Intermittent Fasting in 5 Easy Steps for Women, By Women: The Secret Women's Fasting and Diet Guide to Maximize Weight Loss and Burn Fat

By: Paula Louise

Intermittent Fasting in 5 Easy Steps for Women, By Women: The Secret Women's Fasting and Diet Guide to Maximize Weight Loss and Burn Fat: by Paula Louise. Published by Honest Reads

www.HonestReads.com

© 2018 Honest Reads

All rights reserved. No portion of this book may be reproduced in any form without permission from the publisher, except as permitted by U.S. copyright law. For permissions contact:

hellohonestreads@gmail.com

Introduction

For many women, just the thought of going without food for more than a couple of hours terrifies them. We often worry about the levels of irritability we may encounter from fasting hunger pains; however, the truth is far from this. Typically, women who follow this diet feel fuller, experience fewer mood swings, and end up feeling lighter. Which, in turn, provides them with a more positive outlook on life.

I've struggled with weight nearly my entire life. I was extremely self-conscious of my body and I tried all kinds of diets to change it. I spent hundreds of dollars on the newest weight loss supplements only to find out they didn't work. I nearly gave up until I discovered Intermittent Fasting.

Intermittent Fasting was the key to opening a different world for me. A world where I was happier and healthier. It changed my life so much that I decided to dedicate my time to help other women like me. After hearing countless success stories from my clients, I was inspired to write a book to help even more people.

Honestly, I thought it would be inspiring to read a fasting book written for women, by women. Too many health and fitness books are written by men who just don't understand us. I worked with several other female Intermittent Fasting experts to come up with the most helpful information. I spent months exploring what other books, that were mostly written by men, left out that was important for us. When we finished, we were confident this was the most helpful and motivational Intermittent Fasting book written for women, by women.

Fasting has been practiced by various religions for centuries, so it is not an entirely new concept as some people may think. However, more recently, it is has come to be viewed as a detox and weight loss mechanism. While it is true that fasting can have a detoxification effect, I believe the most rewarding benefit is being able to lose weight and feel better about yourself. Compared to the ancient methods of fasting where people would go days without eating, the modern day Intermittent Fasting options are a tad shorter.

This book will walk you through all you need to know about Intermittent Fasting. From how it works, to how to safely quit fasting after long periods of time. You will learn how to make wiser and healthier choices to improve your overall health and wellness. When you find out what is involved and how Intermittent Fasting works; I am sure you will be eager to begin this diet. Best of luck, I hope you find this book as enjoyable as it was writing it.

Table of Contents

Introduction

Chapter 1. The Medical Science Behind Intermittent Fasting

Chapter 2: Why Intermittent Fasting Stands Out Compared To Other Diets

Chapter 3. Benefits Of Intermittent Fasting

Chapter 4. 5 Easy Steps To Get Started And Stick With Intermittent Fasting

Chapter 5. How To Easily Get Over The 21 Day Hump

Chapter 6. Motivation Tips And Words Of Wisdom

Chapter 7: How To Safely End Your Fast

Chapter 8. Common Issues Women Experience With Intermittent Fasting And How To Overcome Them

Conclusion

Chapter 1. The Medical Science Behind Intermittent Fasting

I honestly believe understanding the medical science behind any diet is crucial to fully comprehending what you're getting yourself into. Some diets have no scientific backing and may be dangerous to your health, whereas others may have decades worth of research. Before changing your lifestyle, always be sure to see if it is medically safe. Thankfully, Intermittent Fasting has countless number of scientific studies that proves it's a safe, effective and beneficial diet.

One of the most common reasons people advocate for Intermittent Fasting is due to the fact that it is well grounded in our evolution. Looking back into our ancestry as humans, our ancestors were primarily hunter-gatherers. Food was not always available to them. If they had a hunt that was not successful, there would be no feasting for potentially days or weeks. On the other hand, if it was a successful hunt, then there would be feasting on meats rich in calories for a short period of time. Like all good things, the feast would end and our ancestors would have to survive again on low-calorie foods such as gathered roots, berries and wild cereals.

Understanding the Science

The lifestyle that our ancestors led caused them to have metabolic and biochemical adaptations through the process of natural selection. This helped maximize the survival capacity of our species in such irregular food supply situations. This is a crucial adaptation that plays a large role in fasting. Our metabolism can be lowered with fasting because our bodies have learned how to preserve energy due to historically infrequent supplies of calories.

Intermittent Fasting has research and studies that support its countless advantages and benefits. Although most of this research has been tested on animals such as lab rats, and not humans, the results can be easily translated over. When humans adapted similar principles, they have shown spectacular progress and results.

Mark Mattson of the National Institute of Ageing (a Federal agency under the United States National Institutes of Health) has done significant amounts of research on fasting. For example, Mattson has conducted several studies which focused on the health advantages of Intermittent Fasting, especially on its effects on the brains and hearts of rodents. His work shows that fasting can help in preserving memory and learning, reducing oxidative stress, and improving bio indicators of diseases.

Mattson has several plausible scientific explanations on why Intermittent Fasting can offer so many health benefits. He cited the hypothesis that whenever we fast, our cells undergo mild stress. During these periods of time, our bodies adapt to the stress by improving our ability to cope with it. Subsequently, it strengthens our bodies and may even allow it to perform better in resisting and fighting off foreign diseases.

When we think of the word "stress," many of us have a negative connotation with it. However, allowing our body and mind to undergo stress brings about significant benefits. An example of this would be working out at the gym. This mere act involves placing stress on our muscular and cardiovascular systems. If you make sure to give your body ample time to recover, it will get stronger. Cells can respond in very much the same way. By consistently and correctly undergoing Intermittent Fasting, our cells can adapt to to these stresses and ultimately become stronger and better.

There were several other clinical studies that Mattson participated in regarding caloric restriction and Intermittent Fasting. In one study, overweight adults who also had mild asthma consumed only 20 percent of their regular caloric intake in between days. The individuals who followed the diet, lost on the average of 8% of their original weight within a two-month period. Not only that, they also had a significant reduction in the indicators of oxidative stress and body swelling.

Mattson was involved with other researchers whom he collaborated with to explore the effects of Intermittent Fasting on continuous energy restriction. For example, he focused a lot of his research on weight loss and various biological indicators of specific health conditions such as: diabetes, cardiovascular diseases, and breast cancer. Mattson and his fellow researchers discovered that Intermittent Fasting was an efficient dietary approach to promote weight loss, improve insulin sensitivity, and other health indicators as well.

Not only that, Mark Mattson also investigated the protective advantages of Intermittent Fasting to our neurons. When you fast for more than 10 hours, your body will quickly tap into its fat storage to sustain energy. Our bodies will then release a surplus of fatty acids or ketones into our bloodstream. When we enter this state, it has been shown that this process helps to protect the learning and memory functionality of our brain. In addition, research has shown that it can also slow down disease progression in the brain.

It is also shown that Intermittent Fasting produces health advantages in itself by simply decreasing the overall intake of calories. That is, if you do not go beyond the recommended daily intake allowance during non-fasting days. On these days, you have to be careful with consuming too many calories because then you may reach a calorie surplus.

Stephen Freedland from Duke University Medical Center in North Caroline actually conducted a study between calorie consumption and progression of diseases. Specifically, Freedland performed a study on the impact of Intermittent Fasting on the growth of prostate cancer in lab mice. Freedland and his research colleagues observed that restriction of calorie intake, without malnutrition, is the only experimental approach that continually showed long-term survival for animal subjects.

The mice were forced into fasting states for at least two days a week for 24-hour periods. During their non-fasting periods, the lab rats, on average, overate and consumed a caloric surplus. Overall their weight did not change at all because the positives gained from fasting netted with the negatives gained from the surplus. Basically, it counteracted whatever the benefits they might have gotten from Intermittent Fasting.

This study showed that even when mice went into fasting, their conditions did not improve if they have overeaten. To see improvement in one's health, Freedland suggests the target should lose weight by decreasing the total amount of calories that they are consuming, rather than concentrating on when those calories are taken. Freedland concluded that when a person does not eat for two-days a week and restricts their diet for the other five days, they can maximize weight loss.

Comparing White Fat and Brown Fats

White fat is used as extra energy storage which can be released, when needed. However, white fat is closely associated with type 2 diabetes and obesity. Brown fat, on the other hand, can burn food fuel and has been shown as a possible solution to prevent metabolic diseases such as obesity.

Recent research has revealed that under certain specific conditions, white fat could be transformed into brown fat which is known as "browning." This has been under investigation as a possible approach towards fighting obesity.

One experiment placed lab rats into two groups. One group was a control group, and the other was an Intermittent Fasting group. The Intermittent Fasting group was not given any food for 24-hours, and then was given food for the next 2-days. The first group (non Intermittent Fasting group) was regularly given food. This experimental setup went on for four months.

Once the test was completed, both groups of lab rats had consumed equal amounts of calories. How? The fasting group was able to catch up with calories on the two days that they were not fasting. At the end of the experiment, the lab rats in the fasting group weighed considerably less compared to the lab rats in the control group, even though they consumed equal amounts of calories.

The researchers also became aware that the insulin sensitivity was increased in the fasting group. Additionally, their metabolism of glucose was more stable in comparison to the control group. Other data this experiment revealed was that the lab rats that fasted had lower amounts of lipid buildup and had healthier livers than their counterparts. Another interesting observation from this experiment is that the fasting group of lab rats had a lower composition of white fat because most of the body fat went into browning.

The researchers conducted another experiment using obese lab rats and discovered that the same types of health advantages occurred just after six weeks of Intermittent Fasting. Additionally, the researchers wanted to understand the metabolic and physiological reasons that allowed for these benefits (especially the conversion of white fat into brown fat). They discovered that the changes in the immune-associated gene channels within fatty cells were one of the sole causes of this adaptation.

Chapter 2: Why Intermittent Fasting Stands Out Compared to Other Diets

Not all diets are created equal. In fact, not all diets are effective, healthy, or even beneficial for you. Some can be seriously detrimental to your wellbeing. I am an advocate for Intermittent Fasting because it brings about a whole bunch of benefits that other diets can't even fathom. This is largely due to the unique concept of "fasting" compared to other conventional diets. For example, other diets solely focus on reducing calorie intake or different types of foods. Fasting, on the other hand, takes on a completely different approach.

You might have heard some negativity around the effects of Intermittent Fasting on women. Some women have reported side effects after trying Intermittent Fasting such as: early menopause, raging PMS, and even losing regular menstrual period. However, this doesn't appear to be the norm. Many women stand by Intermittent Fasting as a very effective form of weight loss regiment. Many believe and experience the many benefits it brings such as: clearing brain fog, boosting fat loss, stabilizing mood swings.

A wide range of conventional diets that require few food choices and stringent calorie restriction usually provide minimal results. Not only that, they can trigger increased feelings of uncontrollable cravings and deprivation. On the other hand, Intermittent Fasting could be as simple as having a late breakfast and lunch, along with early dinners and avoiding late night snacks. Really, it's that simple.

Speed Up Weight Loss and Reduce Aging

In 2011, there was research conducted during the yearly scientific conference by the American College of Cardiology about Intermittent Fasting. They discovered that Intermittent Fasting can trigger a shocking 1,300% increase of HGH (Human Growth Hormones) among women. It's true that both women and men produce HGH but the hormone acts slightly differently in each sex. This is the reason women who are low in HGH have different symptoms that men who are low on it.

The fitness hormone is known as "HGH" plays a critical role in maintaining maximum levels of longevity, fitness, and health. This, in turn, speeds up the weight loss process and stimulates muscle production throughout the body. HGH has an amazing ability to help our bodies lose fat, without compromising muscular development. In fact, many women athletes consider integrating fasting within their fitness regiments because they want to leverage this particular hormone as much as possible.

Not only that, HGH therapy is recommended for women who experience a shortage of it. These therapies increase HGH which, in turn, reduces mature aging, increases youthfulness, and even slow life threatening symptoms. In addition to therapy, doctors prescribe medication to women to curb these symptoms. For example, birth controls, anti depressants etc.

These are all temporary solutions that don't actually address the root cause. On the other hand, Intermittent Fasting has shown a drastic increase of HGH production in women, which may be a natural remedy for these issues.

Reduce Your Unhealthy Sugar Cravings

Research has revealed that, in comparison with regular calorie restriction, Intermittent Fasting is more effective in enhancing insulin resistance and in achieving weight loss. Moreover, those who have successfully activated their fat-burning mode soon discovered their sugar cravings have disappeared.

Eliminating or reducing sugar cravings is especially important for women because studies show that females crave sweets more than males. Lisa A. Eckele from the Florida State University Program in Neuroscience conducted a sugar consumption study on rats. Eckel initially monitored the rats' typical eating patterns with a regular diet where no exercise was allowed. Subsequently, she offered sweetened condensed milk along with the standard diet.

Although both rats consumed the sweetened milk, in addition to their standard diet, the females actually consumed 25% to 20% more calories than the males. Additionally, the females gained 30% more weight compared to 10% more for males. When they were given the opportunity to exercise, it appeared that both males and female reduced their calorie intake. Males cut back to their original intake whereas females only cut back around 20%.

Eckel believes it may be the female hormone estradiol that enhances these sweet cravings. For example, research on human cravings has revealed greater preference for chocolate during menstrual cycles. Unfortunately, it doesn't end there. Over consuming sweets causes you to eat more sweets. This is because sweets will make your blood sugar rise, then dip, which makes you hungry again.

Help Fight Forms of Cancer

Fasting is associated with the prevention and early treatment of breast cancer. A study published in *Cancer Cell*, indicates that a diet similar to fasting basically starves out breast cancer cells. Additionally, it increases the cancer cells' sensitivity to chemotherapy and improves the immune system's chances to fight the tumor.

Regular treatments for these types of cancers such as chemotherapy and radiotherapy, typically reduces immune cells to destroy cancer. Being in a fasting state actually increases the sensitivity of cancer cells to chemotherapy, while reducing the effect on normal cells from the drug's side effects.

The researches forced mice models of breast cancer into a fasting state. This means they were given only 50% of their normal diet, and only 9.7% of it the following 3 days. After 4 days, they were given a normal diet for 10 days before going into another fasting state. This plan showed the reduction in breast cancer cell growth without chemotherapy. It also made cancer cells more sensitive to drugs found in chemotherapy. In a melanoma model, where they fasted and used chemotherapy, there was a 3x reduction in tumor size compared to rats with a standard diet.

Chapter 3. Benefits of Intermittent Fasting

The biggest motivator that convinced me stick with fasting was learning about all the benefits it brings. By understanding what I was working towards, I was able to view my life in the bigger picture. I realized that I'm not only losing weight or looking sexier. I'm drastically improving my health and prolonging my lifespan. Whenever I get discouraged, I always re-read these benefits to remind myself of the bigger picture. To reignite the spark and continue with my fasting journey.

Make Your Skin Glow

Many people that have introduced Intermittent Fasting into their lifestyles have reported positive effects on their skin. In my teenage years, I suffered from several skin issues such as oily skin, acne, and breakouts. When I began to eat my meals for limited hours in a day, my skin improved drastically. But, once I started to eat early breakfasts or have late night meals, I would experience breakouts again. I eventually concluded that the earlier results I gotten were because of fasting. When you give your body extended breaks from routine digestion, it helps kick-start your body's detox mechanism. It also helps your body digest food better and allows it to de-stress. Because of all of this, your skin will begin to glow, and you will naturally reduce skin-related problems.

Improved Breathing

You may not think that poor breathing can affect you until you are faced with a respiratory issue. I struggled for years with shortness of breath. I had my doctor check to see if I had asthma, but the reports didn't show anything. I then began to think that it was my weight that was affecting my breathing. So, with that, I started following various fad diets and ended up feeling sicker. Your life can feel very miserable when you are not able to breathe correctly; I was feeling stuck. I slowly began to cut down on all the dairy and gluten in my diet and started taking vitamin B12 shots. Along with that, I began Intermittent Fasting, and my breathing improved until I got to the point where I no longer suffered from shortness of breath.

Reduce Stress

Free radicals are produced by our bodies when we breathe. A decent and healthy level is fine, as they stimulate repair. However, when our body produces more than it should, it can damage our cells which is called oxidative stress. It is one of the factors for aging skin, wrinkles, and graying hair.

Studies have revealed that Intermittent Fasting may improve the resistance our bodies have to oxidative stress. Oxidative stress is a process that leads to the destruction of essential molecules through reactions with other unstable molecules, such as free radicals. Also, there are more facts and evidence supporting that Intermittent Fasting can help fight against inflammation, which is a common cause of many chronic diseases.

Reduce Inflammation

One of the main reasons for inflammation is excessive free radicals in your body resulting in cellular damage. When our cells' mitochondria's (the powerhouse in our cells that give us energy) are damaged, they begin to release excessive free radicals. These, in turn, result in inflammation and DNA damage. All these problems vanish when you allow your body to be in a fasted state for extended hours.

Fasting helps to control the release of free radicals present in your body. This results in being able to protect your body from inflammation. Those who eat throughout the day are also consuming excessive amounts of salt, which is responsible for excessive bloat. When you practice fasting for prolonged hours, with ample water consumption, you can help to ensure that you never have to face inflammation issues again.

Improve Your Brain's Health

Intermittent Fasting improves processes that are very crucial for our brain health. It can lead to reduced inflammation, reduced oxidative stress, reduced blood sugar levels and increased insulin resistance. It also helps to increase the levels of a brain-driven neurotrophic factor, a brain hormone whose deficiency is linked to depression and other similar problems of the brain.

Repair Your Cells

Fasting can lead to autophagy, which is a cellular process for removal of waste. This entails cells breaking down and metabolizing dysfunctional, broken proteins, which build up in cells over extended periods of time. During this autophagy, your body builds protection against several diseases like Alzheimer's disease and cancer.

CHAPTER 4. 5 EASY STEPS TO GET STARTED AND STICK WITH INTERMITTENT FASTING

I always thought Intermittent Fasting was difficult because of all the rules I had to follow; however, when I actually did it, I found it be pretty easy. You might be confused on where to start or what to even do. Don't worry, we will walk through this journey together. Intermittent Fasting significantly changed my life for the better and I want to help you change yours. That's why I boiled down how to get started with Intermittent Fasting in 5 easy steps.

Incorporating Intermittent Fasting into your lifestyle doesn't need to be complicated. The primary core principle that you need to follow is that you must avoid eating for most of the day and wait to consume the recommended calories during the "feast days" (which could last from three to four days a week).

Many people find this dietary habit uncomfortable. However, this is not a fad diet. It has been proven, through medical research and studies, to be an effective way to easily comply with your dietary needs. Plus, you can make it more fun for yourself.

Many people find this dietary habit more exciting compared to other conventional eating habits, as you can still enjoy bigger servings during your eating days. You will soon realize that this guide supports the principles of a proper diet, and the primary reason to follow it is that you will genuinely enjoy it.

It can be a simple process, that will only take you five steps to get started:

1. Choose a fasting plan that will suit your needs.
2. Count your calories.
3. Count your macronutrients.
4. Follow a meal plan that is effective for you.
5. Exercise while you are fasting.

The last step (step 5) is optional, but the first four steps are crucial to make this diet plan effective and fruitful for your objectives.

Step 1—Choose the fasting plan that suits your needs

In recent years, Intermittent Fasting has become very popular, offering different types of fasting that you can choose from depending on your personal preferences and needs.

Leangains or 16:8

Leangains or 16:8 is the first type of fasting that was developed by Martin Berkhan. This is a plan that was designed mainly for athletes, or for individuals that are working for the specific composition of their bodies. This is a popular choice amongst bodybuilders.

With the Leangains approach, women must go into a fasting period of 16-hours and consume food for the rest of the 8-hours of the day. The fasting begins after you have consumed your last food for the day, and it stops with your first meal.

With this approach to fasting, you should try not to eat or drink anything with calories during the 16 hour window. Things such as sugar-free gum, sugar alternatives, and black coffee are allowed. The Leangains approach recommends skipping breakfast which most people today are already doing.

The Warrior Fasting

The Warrior Fasting is a type of fasting that was popularized with the help of Ori Hofmekler. With this approach, you do not eat for 20-hours every day and then consume one big meal every night. You may choose to have several small meals composed of vegetables, protein, and fruits within a 20-hour period that will lead up to your hearty dinner. This will increase your insulin level that will cause your fasting period to stop.

Hofmekler believes that taking a sizable percentage of our calories in the evening is in accordance with our body composition, which could help us lose fat faster and develop more muscle. However, this claim is often criticized due to the lack of available research.

Other critics say that the Warrior Fasting method can be a challenge to use if your macronutrients need to be worked on. It can be hard to maintain an appetite by consuming the required surplus of protein in one big meal. This approach is recommended for those that enjoy eating one large meal day.

Eat Stop Eat

The Eat Stop Eat approach to Intermittent Fasting was created by Brad Pilon. This is an approach that is both easy to understand and execute. With this approach, you would fast once or twice a week for a 24-hour period. You can start the fasting period whenever you like, but it should last for 24-hours. During this time, you will be encouraged not to eat or drink foods that have calories; you will still be able to drink calorie-free beverages such as tea and coffee.

If you feel that you are not ready to fast for a full 24-hour period, then you can start in a shorter period such as 10-hours then slowly build your way up. After your fasting period, bon apetit the rest of the non-fasting days.

Alternate Day Fasting

Alternate Day Fasting (ADF) is a form of Intermittent Fasting in which you fast and feast in between days. Similar to Warrior Fasting, on your fasting days, you do not strictly fast as you still need to eat at least 20 percent of your Total Daily Energy Expenditure (TDEE), which is around 300-400 calories for women. During your feast days, it would be ideal to eat less than the energy you need to do your usual activities.

ADF is a method to lose weight; you should not increase your consumption of calories to compensate for days that you are taking low calories. ADF makes good sense for those that are sedentary or overweight. However, ADF is not recommended for everyone because it is not advisable for those who are working out as you will need the energy to sustain your training regimen. During minimal calorie periods, you should consume more protein to limit the loss of muscle.

5:2

5:2 means for 5 days a week you would eat normally (maintain your caloric intake, make sure not to overeat!). Then on the other 2 days, you would reduce your caloric intake to a quarter of your maintenance needs. This is typically around 500 calories for women. Feel free to pick any two days of the week you find easiest to commit to. Just keep in mind there should be at least 1 non-fasting day in between the 2 fasting days.

Some women commonly plan to fast on Mondays and Thursdays and only eat 2 to 3 small meals. Then, they would eat "normally" for the remainder of the week. The most important thing to remember on non-fasting days is to not overeat. You need to maintain your calorie intake so that you maintain your weight. If you binge eat on the non-fasting days then you may gain weight if you're at a caloric surplus.

Which Plan Should You Follow?

I personally follow Leangains, which is a workable and straightforward approach for Intermittent Fasting. However, one size does not fit all. It's difficult to say one plan is more effective or better than the other because it's all dependent on your lifestyle. You need to evaluate the context and situation you're currently in and measure it against the available plans. I recommend you try whichever fasting style fits better with your lifestyle.

Step 2—Count Your Calories

Some people believe that you do not need to count calories while you are Intermittent Fasting. There is no truth behind this statement. Regardless of the dietary protocol you choose to follow, counting calories is always essential. If you want to lose weight, you are going to want to keep track of your caloric consumption. The more that you follow the plan, the more likely you gain better results in the long-term.

What is the ideal number of calories for you to consume? There are various methods to determine this. In fact, there are online calculators that you can use. Just Google, "calorie counter calculator."

An easy and straightforward way that you can count your calorie target is to multiply your body weight in kilograms by 40 or 29, respectively, to gain muscles or lose weight. If for example, your weight is 60 kg, you should target to consume at least 1, 740 calories every day to lose weight and 2,400 calories to gain muscle.
Some calculators request that you fill in your weight, activity level, and body fat percentage so you can get the level of lean muscle you have, your basal metabolic rate and your TDEE. Below are the guidelines for your calorie intake:

- To sustain your current weight, consume 100% of your daily expenditure.
- To add more weight, consume 110% of your daily expenditure.
- To lose weight, consume 75% of your daily expenditure.

Step 3—Count Your Macronutrients

You need to be aware that calories and macronutrients are as important as dieting and exercising. It'll be difficult to achieve your fitness goals if you are not paying attention to these components together. Calories are composed of macronutrients that are essential to life. The three primary macronutrients are carbohydrates, fat, and protein.

Generally, these macronutrients contain the following calorie levels:

1 gram of fat = 9 calories
1 gram of carbohydrates = 4 calories
1 gram of protein = 4 calories

It can be almost impossible to keep track of your macronutrients without counting your calories. Certain specific aspects suggest tracking your macros should be a higher priority compared to calorie counting:

- A healthy hormone profile can be promoted by eating sufficient amounts of fat which helps in better nutrient absorption
- You will be able to recover more comfortably from a workout by eating sufficient amounts of carbohydrates
- Improve your muscle development, control hunger, sustain muscle while dieting, and recover from your workouts quicker by eating a sufficient amount of protein.

It is crucial that you keep track of your macros and consume enough amount of fat, protein, and carbohydrates. But, how do you count your macronutrients? You should begin with your protein consumption. If you want to sustain or gain weight, then 1 gram of protein for every pound of body weight is enough. If you are interested in losing fat, research reveals that you must eat around 1 to 1.2 grams of protein for every pound of your body.

Next, you need to figure out your fat consumption. If you want to safely reduce fat, then consume at least 0.2 grams of fat for each pound of body weight every day. To help sustain muscle gain, you need to increase that to 0.3 grams for every pound per day. Finally, for carbohydrates consumption, it simply composes the rest of your caloric requirement for the day, which is between 30 percent and 50 percent of your total daily calories for most people.

Step 4—Follow a Meal Plan that Works for You

The challenging work and effort it will take you to build your best body can easily be impacted by simple things. For example, if you are not following a plan that you can consistently follow, your efforts will be tossed down the train.

That is why it is vital for Intermittent Fasting that you are skilled in meal planning. This is the best way to help ensure that you see the results that you want. A meal plan is merely a plan for the food that you want to eat and when you intend to eat. Keep in mind, that it does not have to be annoying, inconvenient, or restrictive. The ideal meal plan is the contrary. You should plan your meal to be exciting. Do not try to restrain yourself from eating the foods that you love.

If you want to lose weight using Intermittent Fasting, it would be a good idea to eat your food intake in a 6 to 8-hour eating window. You can do this by going 5 to 6 hours after you wake up before taking your meal and your last meal could be two hours before you go to sleep. For example, if you get up at 10 am, have your first meal between 3-4 pm, your second meal between 6-7 pm and your last meal of the day at 10 pm.

If you skip breakfast, this will allow your system to access its stored fat to gain more fuel rather than burning food for energy. This is one of the many reasons why Intermittent Fasting is thought to be a useful tool for weight loss among women. Also, by delaying daily food intake, you can enjoy healthy meals while you stay in your caloric deficit.

You might need a bit of time to get used to skipping breakfast; this is one of the more difficult aspects of integrating Intermittent Fasting into your lifestyle. Eventually, your body will learn to adjust to your fasting period. It will activate its sympathetic mode, and you will be able to feel the hunger blunting effect, improved focus, and alertness.

Drink Coffee While You Fast

When you first get into fasting, you may find it physically and emotionally challenging because your body needs to adapt to the fasting state. I strongly suggest drinking coffee. It will help improve your mood, decrease your cravings, and boost your metabolism. If you are going to gym and working out, then a coffee can also have a positive effect on your stamina and strength.

Coffee tends to have an invigorating effect that can last up to six hours. Even if you exercise later in the day, you can still obtain the benefits from your morning cup of brew. Coffee is also rich in antioxidants and can help to flush out toxins from your body.

What To Eat On Non-Fasting Days

Try keeping your first two meals of the day modest and healthy. It is possible that if you break your fast with a large meal, it can transform your body from your sympathetic mode into parasympathetic mode. This will cause the process of burning fat to shut down which can make you easily tired. This is not ideal mid-morning or early afternoon. A massive meal during the day is not effective in restricting hunger. Make sure that you seek professional advice from your doctor as people's responses to cravings differ from person to person.

Keep in mind that Intermittent Fasting is a way to take enough food and nutrients, and resist hunger without adverse effects on your health. It will also enable you to boost your focus and energy.

Examples of Meals non-fasting days:

Meal No. 1
- Avocado, Apple, Chicken breast, green salad

Meal No. 2
- Can of tuna, apple, 1 tablespoon of olive oil

Meal No. 3.
- Greek yogurt or cottage cheese topped with almonds and berries

Meal No. 4
- Berries and omelet

Meal No. 5
- Whey mixed with almond milk, and fruits

The above example of intermittent meals includes enough protein sources, healthy fat, and fruits. These meals could help you lower your caloric intake, without compromising your mood. Fruits are great in restoring glycogen in your liver, are rich in nutrients, and are easy to digest.

With the glycogen increase in your liver, your body will be able to shift into the anabolic stage and reduce hunger. It is best to include a source of fat in your diets such as whole eggs, olive oil, and nuts. If you decide to keep fat sources at a minimum, you might find yourself feeling hungry relatively soon. Yogurt, fruits, and nuts are an easy choice for your meals that are simple to prepare and don't require cooking.

Step 5—Exercise while You Fast

The fifth step in getting started with Intermittent Fasting is exercise during the fasting period. This is optional as not everyone can workout while they are fasting.

If you do decide to exercise during your fast, your insulin level will decrease, and your body will rely more heavily on its energy reserves. A cool trick is to exercise two hours after you eat. Then your body can depend on the energy from the food you just consumed as your insulin level will increase.

Most people that are into Intermittent Fasting tend to prefer working out in the morning, then break their fasts by consuming a healthy post-exercise meal. Some people also like fasted training while cutting down their meal intake. This helps to burn more fat while they exercise, especially stubborn fat throughout the body.

Chapter 5. How to Easily Get Over The 21 Day Hump

Your first three weeks will be the most challenging in your fasting career. The first couple of times I tried Intermittent Fasting, I had difficulty getting over the 21-day hump. I kept revisiting this diet because I wanted to lose weight and improve my health. I wanted to feel better about myself and get my confidence back. I realized it took 21 days before it starting getting easier. Trust me, after 3 weeks of Intermittent Fasting, it's pretty much downhill from there. This chapter is dedicated to all the tips I followed that helped push me to the 22nd day.

Blend Fasting Into Your Lifestyle

Before you decide to take up fasting, plan your meals. Don't consume meals randomly during these times. This is something that could trigger excessive exertion and result in loss of energy. You want to ensure that your schedule is relaxed so that the sudden change does not negatively affect you. Whatever plan you chose, remember to keep your routine stress-free.

Don't Overeat

I understand that you may find the idea of fasting a bit scary. I understand you may feel like you want to stuff yourself with food after fasting for so long. However, it could be detrimental to your actual progress if you don't focus on the macronutrients. Most dieticians will suggest eating a meal with a lot of healthy fat, lean proteins and plenty of vegetables. You may also choose to include some legumes or even a sweet potato to curb your cravings.

Adding some fruit to your meals can provide your body with some natural sugar, and help to curb your sugar cravings. Fruit that is low-glycemic such as berries can be consumed in moderation. These types of meals can provide you with ample nutrition, so you will be able to carry out your fasting period as smoothly as possible.

Be Prepared

To take on a sudden change in diet, it is vital to make sure that you are well rested and mentally prepared. A person that is emotionally healthy should be able to sail through the initial food cravings that may arise. Additionally, you should make sure that you keep your temptations out of reach. A way that you can do this is to make sure that your kitchen is cleared of all processed foods and sugary drinks. You need to eliminate unhealthy food items right away. When it comes to fasting remember the cliché, "out of sight is out of mind." This is a mantra that can be easily memorized and help you to stay focused on your fasting goals.

Avoid Rigorous Exercises

During your fasting stage, you are not going to want to try and run a 5-mile marathon (I don't recommend it). Instead, you should do light exercise like jogging or yoga. Any high-intensity cardiovascular workout routine during your fasting state may prove difficult for you to maintain, and make you extremely tired. There are passive activities like acupuncture and massages that some nutritionists suggest, which can help increase your blood flow. It also helps to lower your cortisol levels, a hormone that stores fat in the body and can break down your muscles. You want your goals to be: 1. burn fat and 2. store muscle. However, I understand that some of you may be marathon runners. You can still do it, but I recommend you take a break from fasting for at least a couple days before the actual run.

Take Your Multivitamins

Depending on the fasting you choose to do, you may need to take some multivitamin supplements. If you are doing the Leangains or 16:8 fast, you may not need multivitamin supplements. But if you are going to be fasting for more than an 18-hour period, you might want to consider taking them. To help with digesting the multivitamins, I suggest that you take them in liquid form. A regular multivitamin pill, which offers 100% of the daily values, will do the trick. Just be sure to consult with your doctor for further advice.

Hydrate!

Your fasting will go much smoother if you keep yourself hydrated. Typically, there is a tendency to confuse the feelings of thirst for hunger. Many of us will not knowingly eat an extra meal when we are thirsty rather than hungry. This can lead us to overeat during our meals. Given this, it is important to keep yourself hydrated when you are fasting. There is a lot of water present in the foods we eat, but not enough to keep us hydrated. The best way to check whether you are hydrated is to check your urine. If your urine is the color of lemonade, then you should drink up.

Discover Distractions

It may be challenging to not eat while you're starting your fast. Make sure to partake in distracting and fun things. Any pleasurable activity that can keep your mind off your diet works well. A fun distraction would be doing something like treating yourself to a gentle, relaxing massage or pedicure. You can try boosting your mood by putting on a new outfit or walking in the park. Basically, just try to avoid hunger triggers. Going to social gatherings such as parties where there is an abundance of food may be difficult. If you are a foodie, then I would suggest that you stay away from mouth-watering pictures online. Find things to keep your mind busy that will involve keeping your mind off fasting.

Accept Help

Being willing to accept a little help, when needed, will help prevent you from getting overwhelmed. In fact, it might be helpful to consider getting a friend or loved one to take up fasting with you. Additionally, you can try online support groups.

After being a part of so many different Intermittent Fasting groups, I've handpicked a few extremely helpful and supportive ones. Trust me, finding a fantastic group of people going through the same thing as you makes all the difference.

Furthermore, you might want to record daily videos of your progress throughout the fasting to help keep you motivated. Ask your partner for some emotional support when you are going through your fasting. This can help to strengthen your bond between you and your partner. It can be very comforting to have someone else share your weight loss goals while making your relationship stronger in the process.

Don't Get Stressed

Ladies, you do not need to weigh yourself every day. You should avoid activities that bring you stress and just stick to your diet plan. Trust me, you'll lose weight if you remain consistent and follow the guidelines. I understand you'll be anxious to check your weight to see if there's any progress but limit these checks to once a month.

If you get stressed, your cortisol levels may shoot up, which in turn will strip you of your mental peace. If you want to gain the best results, then I would suggest that you consider trying yoga or meditation. Try to involve deep breathing exercises as much as possible to calm your nerves and relax your body. Try to avoid too strenuous activities. You will need to conserve your energy while you are fasting, so that you are able to function throughout the day. Do not fret over your progress, if you find yourself initially struggling, just remember that it will get better and easier as time goes by.

Avoid The Victory Binge

When you weigh yourself after a month and see that you successfully lost weight, you should celebrate and reward yourself. Take a day or two and just enjoy your new beautiful body. Appreciate and indulge in the feeling of being just a tad lighter. Just keep in mind, if you don't want to fall back to your old diet pattern then I suggest you don't fall into the "victory binge" trap. Please just remember to eat food in moderation. Make sure that your meals are full of fiber and non-cruciferous vegetables so you feel full throughout the day. Limit yourself to 5-ounces of wine or 1 can of beer. Savor your treats and enjoy each and every mouthful—keeping it all in moderation is the key to many things in life! Remember the cliché, "Too much of a good thing is not good."

Chapter 6. Motivation Tips and Words of Wisdom

I'll admit it, I needed a lot of motivation. The reason I quit Intermittent Fasting the first couple of times was because I wasn't motivated enough. Trust me, it's a crucial part of being able to reap the benefits of this diet. It's going to get challenging and sometimes it's the only thing that keeps you going. I dedicated a chapter to motivation and words of wisdom to help you understand your reasons and your "why."

Find Your Why

In order to stay motivated and stick with Intermittent Fasting, you need to ask yourself why losing weight is important to you. Do you want to get ready for summer and swimsuit weather? Do you need to do this for health reasons? Do you want to feel good about yourself? Do you want to look better? Go beyond aesthetic reasons because that's only temporary. Make sure you do a bit of searching in your mind to truly find a more permanent reason to motivate you. Perhaps you want to live longer to see your grandchildren? Or to live longer to see more of the world.

I understand, finding a more permanent motivation is not so simple. I have a tip on how you can start your search though. Begin with aesthetic motivational reasons and list them down on a piece of paper. Use these as a baseline to help you to get going. Write down what motivates you and pin it near your mirror so that you can be reminded. Eventually you'll be able to tack on more and more motivational reasons to the list. On the days you are feeling down from fasting, look at your list to lift your spirits and stick to your plan.

Work on Your Short-Term Process Goals

Aside from your ultimate goal, you should also try and work on your short-term process goals. Try not to focus too much on losing 10 pounds after three months. You should determine how you can achieve it. Process goals could mean giving up unhealthy food, setting up your fasting schedule, counting your calories, and more. Make these goals within your reach, and once you have achieved them, it will serve your motivation to keep you going forward.

A tip is to make SMART goals, which stands for Specific, Measurable, Attainable, Realistic, and Time-bound. For example, "I will stop snacking on chips on the weekdays for the next 5 weeks." Make sure your goals follow the SMART guideline to keep your motivation and progress up.

Establish Realistic Goals

In losing weight through Intermittent Fasting, among the first thing you need to achieve is to set realistic goals for yourself. You do not want to set unrealistic goals as this will lead to failure. Intermittent Fasting is a gradual process to help you to lose weight slowly but surely. Losing at least one to two pounds per week is healthy and achievable. Leveling your expectations will help provide you with that added motivation to keep going.

If you expect too much from Intermittent Fasting, like losing 5 pounds a week, you will just be setting yourself up for failure. When your goals are unrealistic and too difficult to achieve, it will demotivate you and you'll just end up quitting. Therefore, please remember to be practical with your goals and expectations.

Using Apps to Keep Track of Your Progress

Being able to keep tabs on your progress is an extremely useful tool to help keep you motivated. For instance, you can make use of the many available apps to see how much time you have fasted, and keep track of your progress.

When you get cravings, just open your app to see how many hours of fasting you accomplished. It'll keep you motivated because you won't want to spoil all your hard work. Your body will typically go into a "burning fat mode" between 12 and 16 hours into fasting. If you're already on your 14th hour, the tracker will motivate you to keep going for a 2 additional hours. You may even gain more motivation if you have an app that averages your weekly fasting. You can keep track of your daily averages which can motivate you to fast even longer on certain days, if your body permits. It'll be like a game where you try to beat your personal high score. Additionally, checking your app throughout the day could be the ideal distraction you need to get rid of your cravings.

Be Your Personal Coach

You are the best person to motivate yourself. You can program your mind to think precisely what you want it to think. You need to drive yourself by positively reinforcing your efforts and reminding yourself of your motivational reasons. Look at yourself in the mirror and say to your reflection (out loud) that you can overcome your food cravings and that you are doing this for your health. Each day, you can program your mind and body to become an incredible fat burning machine. When you use these self-motivational methods, your brain will believe everything you tell yourself. If you think you are going to fail, you will inevitably fail. But, if you genuinely think that you will succeed, you will succeed!

Follow the Five-Second Rule

Mel Robbins popularized the five-second rule as a motivational trick. In her book, she describes it by counting from five to one and then doing whatever you need to do, immediately. Using this simple motivational trick has helped thousands of people make life-changing transformations, not only regarding their health but also in their careers, relationships, finances and more.
When you want to begin fasting, just countdown from five to one and begin. This can easily empower and motivate you!

Be Willing to Forgive Yourself

Don't forget, Intermittent Fasting is not a walk in the park. You may realize it's not as easy as people make it out to be. There are going to be times when you slip up and make a mistake. Perhaps you choose to attend a birthday party, and in the process, you ate delicious food instead of sticking to your fasting schedule. That's absolutely fine. Just remember, do not beat yourself up about it because this is normal and you're only human. Instead of punishing yourself, realize the mistake, and immediately get back on track and move forward.

Make sure, after your eating mishap, to have a light and healthy meal the next time you can eat. Never starve yourself just because you accidentally had a feast the day before. We all make mistakes—remember, "to err is human," especially when it comes to sticking to our diets. We should try to learn from our mistakes. When you are too hard on yourself, you may begin to think that Intermittent Fasting is not effective because you eventually give up on it. Avoid falling into this trap as it will only lead to emotional overeating. Stick with it.

Chapter 7: How to Safely End Your Fast

Many women ask me, "how can I safely stop Intermittent Fasting?" Whether you fasted for months or years, it's important to stop the healthy way. You want to reduce as much stress and shock to your body as possible.

Depending on what type of fast you decided to do will determine the best way for you to come off of it. If you're fasting for health reasons, the best way to come off a fast is slowly and steadily. I recommend you start by eating bone broth. Bone broth is filled with collagen that will help you absorb electrolytes, plus it plays a vital role in your gut health by producing gelatin to protect the lining. Additionally, bone broth contains glycine that helps to build up RNA and DNA, so your body can rebuild cells. You can also use a tablespoon of apple cider vinegar with a dash of sea salt and cinnamon in hot water. The apple cider will increase mineral and vitamin intake.

If you are coming off a fast for fat loss reasons it is best to do so by using a bit of MCT oil—this will by pass through the liver and go directly into the bloodstream. It will give your body a quick infusion of fats that will get your body to use the fat as a source of energy.

There aren't many studies done on how to break Intermittent Fasting after a prolonged period of time. The above instructions are just recommendations that I came up with based on my experiences. I believe bone broth, apple cider vinegar, and MCT oil are all extremely helpful to easing back into a regular eating routine.

Chapter 8. Common Issues Women Experience with Intermittent Fasting and How to Overcome Them

I love to be prepared, especially whenever I start something new. It's the positive feeling of being able to take control, as much as possible, of the situation I'm in. That is why I decided to add this chapter to the book. It was beyond helpful for me to learn the common problems I might encounter with Intermittent Fasting. This allows me to proactively avoid or overcome them, which makes everything much easier.

Figuring Out If Intermittent Fasting Is For You

Intermittent Fasting is not a one size fits all. You need to make sure your lifestyle and health allows it. Many people start without realizing it's nearly impossible for them to maintain it.

It is important that you check with your doctor to find out if this diet is right for you, especially if you have any underlying medical conditions. If you are already suffering from a serious ailment or if you are pregnant, it is even more vital to consult with your physician before you start this type of fasting. It is always a good idea to find professional help from someone such as a nutritionist, a fitness coach, or your physician, so you are rightly guided. It is essential that you are aware of what is right for you rather than guessing.

This will also help to ensure that there are no health consequences, especially for those that have pre-existing conditions. It is always better to be safe than sorry. If you have been going through a lot of mental and physical stress lately, then it's advisable that you first work on reducing your stress levels before starting with Intermittent Fasting.

When you reach a point where you feel that your mind and body can handle Intermittent Fasting, you can begin.

Trust The Process

We have been conditioned to feel that we need to eat every few hours. This is what causes many people to question the legitimacy of Intermittent Fasting. "Am I starving my body?", "Shouldn't I be fed all the time?" Or "Is skipping breakfast a good idea? I mean, after all, I thought it was the most important meal of the day." If you find yourself thinking along these lines, immediately remind yourself that these statements are not accurate. For a refresher, go back to the beginning of the book. You need to stick and commit to your plan, no matter what. As with any diet or fasting, it requires a certain amount of time before it starts working. It's hard to see daily changes, so stick with a biweekly or even monthly result review. Don't get discouraged if you don't see any changes day to day. Trust me, it works if you follow the plan.

Snacking Is a Big Problem

Have you ever noticed how much we consume in just snacks, even when we are not hungry? Snacking for most people is more of a habit than a necessity. Many of us will choose to snack on fried or processed foods which only makes it more difficult for our body to lose weight. So, in order to be successful at Intermittent Fasting, you need to filter out all the unhealthy junk food snacks right away.

Once your body begins to adjust itself to extended periods of fasting, your natural insulin levels, as well as the hormone cycle, begin to function more effectively. When you find it easier to control your urge to snack, you will notice how light your body will start to feel.

Don't Dive Right In

People tend to dive head first into Intermittent Fasting and fail. You need to ease into it slowly to make sure your body can adjust safely. Begin with cutting all kinds of snacks from your daily routine. If you're hungry, drink a few cups of plain black coffee, which has no caloric value. It'll fill you up and reduce your hunger. Intermittent Fasting requires gradual transition for it to be more effective. During the first couple of weeks try to adapt by trying a high-fat diet first, then you can slowly add fasting hours and days into your schedule. For example, you can make one day your fasting day and see how that feels. If you get used to it, try making it two days, until you are comfortable fasting at least three times a week.

If you are used to having breakfast, abruptly eliminating it may not seem possible. Instead, you may want to try delaying when you have your breakfast a bit every day. You can begin by having it at 10 am and adjusting the rest of the meals within the next 8-hour eating period. Trust me, you do not have to eat breakfast early in the morning. You can eat it later in the day and maintain your fasted state for longer. If you get too excited about fasting, and change your entire lifestyle immediately, there is a good chance you won't be able to maintain it.

Don't Give in! Stay Distracted

Many people give into cravings when they start fasting. You need to remember to stick with the diet and ignore all your food desires. A trick is to sip on your favorite hot beverages (minus the added sugar). If you add milk to any of your beverages, make sure it is low-calorie skimmed milk.

You may sip on different types of green tea, herbal tea, plain black coffee, etc. If you find it hard to sip on unsweetened beverages, then you may add a few drops of Stevia for some sweetness. However, sugar consumption is a complete no-no, as it is known to add a lot of empty calories which then gets stored in your body in the form of fat. When you consume it in excess, it is likely to enter your bloodstream, putting you at high risk of developing diabetes. Sipping on low-calorie drinks can help you to be distracted away from wanting to snack and keep you refreshed.

Stay Focused

No matter what, try not to cave in! Remember your goal and motivation whenever you feel like giving up. You may have taken up Intermittent Fasting to lose weight, to detox your body or to improve your health. You need to make a point of reminding yourself of your objective with this fast. An excellent way to help you to stay focused is to write down the reasons why you have chosen to fast. Read this each day before you begin you begin your day. By doing this ritual, you are going to program yourself to concentrate on what you are aiming to achieve rather than caving in.

On the occasions that you fail to keep up with the fast, don't waste time beating yourself up about it. It is okay not to have the complete willpower. However, steer yourself in the direction that will lead you to get back on track without wasting time dwelling on your mistakes. Start the next day fresh and know that you can achieve whatever goals you set for yourself.

You will soon discover how easy it can be to stay motivated when you have a support group. You'll also be able to pick up some tips and learn from others.

Tone Down Your Workouts

It's often that potency requires minimalism. Many women who follow Intermittent Fasting over train and end up exhausting themselves. They blame how terribly their feeling entirely on their fast and end up quitting.

They rarely think working out at a very high intensity for extended periods of time is the main culprit. When you exert too much effort (intensity) than what your body can currently handle, under a fasting state, you run the risk of burning out, becoming sick, or even injured. Even with the right intensity, working out significantly longer than your body can handle runs the same kind of risk. The trick is to train at the correct workout intensity and duration. So how do we know what the correct workout intensity and duration is? You would feel very light-headed, very tired and weak or have prolonged muscle soreness—during or after your workouts if you over-train.

Use the talk test to see if you are exercising at a moderate intensity. If you can carry on a normal conversation while you are working out, albeit, with some difficulty, that's moderate.

You can focus your training by prioritizing compound exercises such as those that involve most major muscle groups to execute the movements. Examples of these would be burpees, which recruit most of your major muscle groups.

Another way you can prioritize your exercises is to choose those that utilize the large muscle groups, particularly legs. Why? The bigger the muscles, the more calories are required to contract them. That is why doing 1,000 crunches aren't enough to get you fit, but running daily for at least 30 minutes, which involves the biggest muscle group (the legs), can help.

During your first two weeks of following Intermittent Fasting, avoid exercise so you can feel how Intermittent Fasting can affect you. Once your body has a chance to get used to the change, there is a significant chance your workouts will be more effective. Start off slow, during this crucial adaptation stage, it is ideal to do some yoga or brisk walking. After this, start adding short jump roping and sprinting sessions to see how you feel.

Monitor Your Hormonal Health

Intermittent Fasting can impact your hormonal health which could affect the balance of your menstrual cycle. There are instances where the slightest changes in our stress-level, toxin exposure, environment, health, and even diet can lead to a hormonal imbalance, potentially leading to more diet issues.

It is crucial that you have the state of your hormones checked before you even begin, as many women don't. If you are already dealing with hormonal imbalance, addressing this issue will have to be prioritized over the fasting plan.

Eating Fat is Acceptable

Many women are scared of eating fats because they think it's the reason for their weight problem. It's not true! Consuming nutrition fats is important, especially when you get into fasting. Examples of healthy fats are grass-fed dairy products, olive oil, avocado oil, eggs, butter, nuts, coconut oil and fat from naturally raised livestock. Once you are used to these foods, you can be sure that you will get enough calories and nutrients in your day before going into fast.

When changing into a high-fat diet, you can ensure that your fasting periods are comfortable, safe and stress-free. By lowering your level of carbs and adding more fat, you can better stabilize your blood sugar levels.

Without the added glucose from your food intake, the stress hormone—the cortisol—will be activated. If you are hungry now, your body will experience stress. But, when following a high-fat diet protocol and once your body has become adjusted to the fat; your blood sugar level will not drop, and the stressor will not exist because your body will not depend on glycogen for energy.

Our bodies know how to run on fats (both stored body fat and dietary fats) rather than depending on the next food intake. Now, not only will you get rid of cravings, but you will also have less stress. And as I mentioned in an earlier part of this book, hormonal imbalance is one of the reasons why Intermittent Fasting can be difficult for women as the body develops cortisol as a response to stress. By choosing to add diverse food and adding high fats to your diet, you can reduce stress.

Don't Starve

Some women may not find Intermittent Fasting effective because they are trying to do it on a strict diet. Keep in mind, that starving yourself is not the primary objective of Intermittent Fasting as it will ultimately lead you to binge eating. During your eating days, you need to eat foods that are high in nutrients with sufficient amount of calories.

Don't Make Weight Loss Your Primary Objective

Millions of people around the world have succeeded in changing their body composition with Intermittent Fasting. Intermittent Fasting is a useful tool for reducing body fat, getting leaner, and losing weight. Women should not do Intermittent Fasting for a get skinny quick scheme. Intermittent Fasting is not some magic pill. It takes commitment and time.

Besides helping you to lose unwanted fat, Intermittent Fasting is a dietary art that offers exciting benefits for your health. For its effects to be long-lasting, you need to have the proper mindset. As a woman, you should look to discover the higher purpose of this dietary change.

It Just Might Not Be For You

Lastly, it just might not be for you. Intermittent Fasting is not for everyone. If you feel dizzy, tired, weak, and miserable, then stop pushing yourself. You need to listen to your body and pay attention to how you feel. If you are absolutely not enjoying it then you need to listen to your body and do what is right for you.

Conclusion

Thanks for downloading my book. I genuinely hope you found it helpful. If you read its entirety, then you pretty much know all there is to know about Intermittent Fasting.

If you decide to give Intermittent Fasting a try, the next step is to set up a plan to safely integrate it into your life. Use this book as a tool to help guide you whenever you need. Follow the steps and use the motivation tips to keep you getting closer to your goals.

Incorporating Intermittent Fasting into your life is going help you lose weight in no time. I wish you the best of luck in making positive, healthy changes in your life.

Happy Fasting!

www.ingramcontent.com/pod-product-compliance
Lightning Source LLC
Chambersburg PA
CBHW031514210526
45464CB00007B/2905